THE NEW CHRONIC LYMPHOCYTIC LEUKEMIA DIET

Learn How to Manage CLL, Strengthen Your Immune System, Eliminate Inflammation, and Promote a Healthier Gut

Michael Slowick, RDN

COPYRIGHT PAGE

herein, no promises are made regarding its completeness or accuracy. Any statements made by sales employees or representatives, whether verbal or written, do not constitute extended or implied guarantees.Chapter 1: Introduction to Chronic Lymphocytic Leukemia (CLL) and Diet

Table of Contents

SAVORY RECIPES AND MEAL IDEAS FOR SNACK

CHAPTER I: CHRONIC LYMPHOCYTIC LEUKEMIA (CLL)

Chronic lymphocytic leukemia (CLL) is a type of blood cancer. It's the most common form of leukemia in adults. It happens when healthy white blood cells (lymphocytes) in your bone marrow mutate, or change, into cancerous cells that multiply and crowd out healthy blood cells and platelets.

CLL typically affects people aged 65 and older, but it can affect people starting at age 30. You can have chronic lymphocytic leukemia without having symptoms. Most people learn they have CLL after having blood tests as part of routine physical examinations.

Currently, healthcare providers don't have routine treatments to cure chronic lymphocytic leukemia. During the past 10 years, providers have developed treatments that put CLL into remission. (Remission means you don't have symptoms and signs of CLL.) These treatments are helping people with CLL live longer.

How common is this condition?

Chronic lymphocytic leukemia is one of the most common types of leukemia in adults. It affects about 5 in 100,000 people in the U.S. The American Cancer Society estimates about 18,700 people will be diagnosed with CLL in 2023. By comparison, more than 238,000 people will be diagnosed with lung cancer in 2023 (one of the most common cancers overall).

Types of chronic lymphocytic leukemia

You may develop CLL in your B-cells or T-cells, which are white blood cells (lymphocytes):

B lymphocytes (B-cells) make antibodies. Antibodies are proteins that target viruses, bacteria and cancer cells, among other foreign intruders.

T lymphocytes (T-cells) control your body's immune system response. T-cells directly attack and destroy abnormal cells, including cancer cells.

Nearly all people with CLL have B-cell chronic lymphocytic leukemia. There's a related condition that affects T-cells called T-cell prolymphocytic leukemia (PLL). People with T-cell PLL develop symptoms more quickly than people who have B-cell CLL.

Causes and Risk Factors of CLL

Causes

Doctors aren't certain what starts the process that causes chronic lymphocytic leukemia. What's known is that something happens to cause changes (mutations) in the DNA of blood-producing cells. A cell's DNA contains the instructions that tell the cell what to do. The changes tell the blood cells to produce abnormal, ineffective lymphocytes.

Beyond being ineffective, these abnormal lymphocytes continue to live and multiply when healthy lymphocytes would die. The abnormal lymphocytes accumulate in the blood and certain organs, where they cause complications. They may crowd healthy cells out of the bone marrow and interfere with blood cell production.

Doctors and researchers are working to understand the exact mechanism that causes chronic lymphocytic leukemia.

Risk factors

Factors that may increase the risk of chronic lymphocytic leukemia include:

Your age: On average, people are 71 years old when they're diagnosed.

Your race: White people are more likely to develop chronic lymphocytic leukemia than are people of other races.

Family history of blood and bone marrow cancers: A family history of chronic lymphocytic leukemia or other blood and bone marrow cancers may increase your risk.

Exposure to chemicals: Certain herbicides and insecticides, including Agent Orange used during the Vietnam War, have been linked to an increased risk of chronic lymphocytic leukemia.

A condition that causes excess lymphocytes: Monoclonal B-cell lymphocytosis (MBL) causes an increased number of one type of lymphocyte (B cells) in the blood. For a small number of people with MBL, the condition may develop into chronic lymphocytic leukemia. If you have MBL and also have a family history of chronic lymphocytic leukemia, you may have a higher risk of developing cancer.

CHAPTER II: SYMPTOMS OF CLL

You can have chronic lymphocytic leukemia without symptoms. It may take months to years before you notice CLL symptoms. Common symptoms include:

Fatigue. CLL affects your red blood cells, causing anemia. Fatigue is a common anemia symptom.

Fever. Fever is a sign of infection. CLL affects healthy white blood cells, increasing your risk of infections.

Swollen lymph nodes in your neck, underarm, groin or stomach.

Night sweats.

Unexplained weight loss.

Pain or a sense of fullness under your ribs. CLL may affect your liver or spleen. Cancerous white blood cells in your liver and/or spleen can make those organs grow.

Complications

Chronic lymphocytic leukemia may cause complications such as:

Frequent infections: If you have chronic lymphocytic leukemia, you may experience frequent infections that can be serious. Sometimes infections happen because your blood doesn't have enough germ-fighting antibodies (immunoglobulins). Your doctor might recommend regular immunoglobulin infusions.

A switch to a more aggressive form of cancer. A small number of people with chronic lymphocytic leukemia may develop a more aggressive form of cancer called diffuse large B-cell lymphoma. Doctors sometimes refer to this as Richter's syndrome.

Increased risk of other cancers: People with chronic lymphocytic leukemia have an increased risk of other types of cancer, including skin cancer and cancers of the lung and the digestive tract.

Immune system problems: A small number of people with chronic lymphocytic leukemia may develop an immune system problem that causes the disease-fighting cells of the immune system to mistakenly attack the red blood cells (autoimmune hemolytic anemia) or the platelets (autoimmune thrombocytopenia).

Diagnosis

Blood tests

Tests and procedures used to diagnose chronic lymphocytic leukemia include blood tests designed to:

Count the number of cells in a blood sample: A complete blood count may be used to count the number of lymphocytes in a blood sample. A high number of B cells, one type of lymphocyte, may indicate chronic lymphocytic leukemia.

Determine the type of lymphocytes involved: A test called flow cytometry or immunophenotyping helps determine whether an increased number of lymphocytes is due to chronic lymphocytic leukemia, a different blood disorder or your body's reaction to another process, such as infection.

If chronic lymphocytic leukemia is present, flow cytometry may also help analyze the leukemia cells for characteristics that help predict how aggressive the cells are.

Analyze lymphocytes for genetic changes: A test called fluorescence in situ hybridization (FISH) examines the chromosomes inside the cancerous lymphocytes to look for changes. Doctors sometimes use this information to determine your prognosis and help choose a treatment.

Other tests

In some cases, your doctor may order additional tests and procedures to aid in diagnosis, such as:

Tests of your leukemia cells that look for characteristics that could affect your prognosis

Bone marrow biopsy and aspiration

Imaging tests, such as computerized tomography (CT) and positron emission tomography (PET)

CHAPTER III: DISEASE PROGRESSION AND STAGING

Healthcare providers use cancer staging systems to develop treatment plans and prognoses (expected outcome). Providers stage CLL with two similar staging systems. The Rai staging system categorizes CLL by the likelihood the condition will get worse and require treatment. The Binet system stages CLL by how much the condition has spread throughout your body.

Rai staging system

The Rai staging system categories are:

Low risk (formerly known as Rai stage 0): You have lymphocytosis and abnormal white blood cells in your blood and/or bone marrow.

Intermediate risk (formerly known as Rai stage I or stage II): You have lymphocytosis, enlarged lymph nodes and an enlarged spleen and/or liver.

High risk (formerly known as Rai Stage III): You have anemia or thrombocytopenia.

Binet staging system

The Binet staging system uses information about your blood cell and platelet count and the number of areas in your body with swollen lymph nodes. Binet staging system categories are:

Stage A: You don't have anemia (low red blood cells) or low platelet levels, but you have swollen lymph nodes in at least two areas in your body. For example, you have swollen lymph nodes in your neck and groin.

Stage B: There are swollen lymph nodes in three areas of your body, liver or spleen, but you don't have anemia and your platelet levels are normal.

Stage C: You have anemia, as well as swollen lymph nodes, in three or more areas of your body.

Some people with cancer feel intimidated or unnerved by systems that seem to reduce their condition to a formula of numbers and letters. Your providers understand why you may feel this way. If you're confused or concerned by what you're hearing, ask your provider to explain how the cancer staging system works in your situation.

Treatment Strategies

How is chronic lymphocytic leukemia treated?

Treatment varies based on your symptoms and test results. For example, if you have early-stage CLL, your healthcare provider may opt for watchful waiting (active surveillance).

In watchful waiting, providers hold off on treatment while carefully monitoring your overall health, symptoms and test results.

Providers also consider genetic test results. For example, certain genetic changes mean your condition is likely to get worse sooner rather than later or typical CLL treatments won't be as effective.

Common CLL treatments include targeted therapy and chemotherapy. Providers may use radiation therapy to ease CLL symptoms. Each treatment type may cause different side effects. Your provider will outline specific treatment benefits, side effects and potential long-term complications.

Targeted therapy

This treatment works by targeting or focusing on cancer cells. In chronic lymphocytic leukemia, treatments keep cancerous white blood cells from growing. Some targeted treatments destroy the cells without hurting healthy cells or platelets. Specific treatments or medication may include:

Bruton's tyrosine kinase (BTK) inhibitor therapy: This treatment blocks the enzymes that cause B-cells to develop into excess white blood cells. Examples include ibrutinib (Imbruvica®), acalabrutinib (Calquence®) and zanubrutinib (Brukinsa ®).

BCL2 inhibitor therapy: Venetoclax (Venclexta®) blocks BCL2, a protein found on leukemia cells, including CLL cells. This treatment can destroy leukemia cells or make them more sensitive to other cancer drugs.

Monoclonal antibody therapy: This treatment is a type of immunotherapy. Monoclonal antibodies are lab-made antibodies that block cancer cell growth or destroy cancerous cells. Examples of monoclonal antibody therapy medications include rituximab (Rituxan®) and obinutuzumab (Gazyva®).

Chemotherapy

Your healthcare provider may use chemotherapy as an initial treatment for chronic lymphocytic leukemia. Common chemotherapy drugs for CLL include:

Fludarabine(Fludara®).

Chlorambucil (Leukeran®).

Cyclophosphamide (Cytoxan®).

Bendamustine (Treanda®).

Immunotherapy

This treatment works by restoring or strengthening your immune system so it can do more to kill cancerous cells or slow down cancerous cell growth.

Providers may use the immunotherapy drug lenalidomide (Revlimid®) to treat chronic lymphocytic leukemia that hasn't responded to chemotherapy, CLL that's come back (recurrent CLL) or CLL that's getting worse.

Medical researchers are evaluating chimeric antigen receptor (CAR-T) therapy for people with CLL that hasn't responded to standard treatment.

Bone marrow transplant: A bone marrow transplant, also known as a stem cell transplant, uses strong chemotherapy drugs to kill the stem cells in your bone marrow that are creating diseased lymphocytes. Then healthy adult blood stem cells from a donor are infused into your blood, where they travel to your bone marrow and begin making healthy blood cells.

As new and more-effective drug combinations have been developed, bone marrow transplant has become less common in treating chronic lymphocytic leukemia. Still, in certain situations this may be a treatment option.

Supportive care

Your doctor will meet with you regularly to monitor any complications you may experience. Supportive care measures may help prevent or relieve any signs or symptoms.

Supportive care may include:

Cancer screening: Your doctor will evaluate your risk of other types of cancer and may recommend screening to look for signs of other cancers.

Vaccinations to prevent infections: Your doctor may recommend certain vaccinations to reduce your risk of infections, such as pneumonia and influenza.

Monitoring for other health problems. Your doctor may recommend regular checkups to monitor your health during and after treatment for chronic lymphocytic leukemia.

Impact of CLL on Nutrition and Dietary Needs

Chronic lymphocytic leukemia (CLL) can impact nutrition and dietary needs due to its effects on the body and the treatments involved. Here are some aspects to consider:

Reduced Appetite: CLL and its treatments can lead to a decreased appetite, nausea, and changes in taste or smell, making it challenging to consume adequate nutrients. It's essential to focus on nutrient-dense foods when appetite is low.

Weight Loss: Some individuals with CLL may experience unintentional weight loss due to factors such as decreased appetite, metabolic changes, or the disease's impact on the body's ability to absorb nutrients. Maintaining a healthy weight is important for overall well-being and immune function.

Nutrient Deficiencies: CLL and its treatments can affect the absorption and utilization of certain nutrients, leading to deficiencies. For example, chemotherapy drugs may interfere with the body's ability to absorb nutrients like vitamin B12, folate, and iron. Nutritional supplements or adjustments to the diet may be necessary to address these deficiencies.

Immune Function: Proper nutrition is crucial for maintaining a healthy immune system, especially for individuals with CLL who may have compromised immune function due to the disease or its treatment. Eating a balanced diet rich in vitamins, minerals, antioxidants, and protein can support immune health and help reduce the risk of infections.

Hydration: Some CLL treatments, such as chemotherapy, can cause dehydration as a side effect. It's important to stay well-hydrated by drinking plenty of fluids, such as water, herbal teas, and electrolyte-replenishing drinks, to support overall health and prevent complications.

Dietary Restrictions: Depending on the individual's condition and treatment plan, there may be specific dietary restrictions or recommendations to follow. For example, some medications may interact with certain foods or supplements, and precautions may be needed to prevent complications.

Gastrointestinal Symptoms: CLL and its treatments can cause gastrointestinal symptoms such as diarrhea, constipation, or mucositis (inflammation of the mucous membranes). Modifying the diet to include easily digestible foods, fiber-rich foods for constipation, and avoiding irritating foods can help manage these symptoms.

Bone Health: Some CLL treatments, such as corticosteroids or chemotherapy, can increase the risk of osteoporosis or bone loss. Adequate intake of calcium, vitamin D, magnesium, and other nutrients essential for bone health is important. Weight-bearing exercises and lifestyle modifications may also be recommended to support bone health.

Overall, maintaining a well-balanced diet tailored to individual needs and addressing any nutritional deficiencies or challenges that arise is essential for managing CLL and supporting overall health and well-being. Consulting with a registered dietitian or healthcare provider knowledgeable about oncology nutrition can provide personalized guidance and support.

CHAPTER IV: ROLE OF DIET IN MANAGING CLL

Many factors influence the development of illnesses like cancer. While cancer can never be fully prevented, research suggests nutrition may play a role. A 2021 study found an association between regularly eating highly processed foods and the odds of developing CLL.

The goal of nutrition during CLL treatment is to help:

Support your immune system

Maintain muscle strength

Ease the side effects of cancer treatment

Reduce inflammation

Maintain a healthy weight

Protect against other health conditions

Focusing on a healthy diet may help support your health during cancer treatment and recovery. There is no specific diet plan recommended for CLL treatment. Instead, most recommendations focus on supporting your overall health with nutritious foods.

Most important during cancer treatment is to focus on eating enough food to prevent unintentional weight loss and malnutrition. Research suggests poor nutrition during cancer recovery increases the risk for negative outcomes.2 Preventing malnutrition and eating enough food helps to improve survival and better health after treatment.

Your healthcare team may provide specific diet recommendations based on your health history and treatment plan. Still, these tips offer information about general guidance for diet and CLL.

The diet plan for CLL focuses on short- and long-term goals. For example, diet recommendations that focus on managing the side effects of chemotherapy will last during medical treatment and while side effects last.

Manage side effects

Treatment side effects may make it difficult to get enough calories and protein.

Side effects of CLL treatments such as chemotherapy include:

nausea

vomiting

diarrhea

constipation

dry or sore mouth and throat (mucositis)

loss of appetite

loss of sense of taste and smell

difficulty chewing or swallowing

Ask your doctor how to manage these side effects so you can still get the nutrition you need to keep your body strong. A diet of soft foods that are easier to chew and swallow can help manage many of these side effects.

Examples of soft foods include:

pureed and strained soups containing lots of vegetables and beans

peanut butter and jelly sandwiches or other soft sandwiches

minced chicken or fish in a sauce

milkshakes or smoothies made with dairy, tofu, soy milk, or yogurt

white rice

omelets or egg scrambles

pureed fruits, like apple sauce or mashed bananas

oatmeal with stewed fruits

Depending on your symptoms, you may need to make certain dietary changes.

For example, if you're experiencing taste changes, adding flavorful additions to meals, such as herbs and spices, may help. Not only can herbs and spices make foods more palatable if you're experiencing changes in taste or smell, but they're also rich in vitamins, minerals, and antioxidants.

However, adding herbs and spices to meals may not suit everyone. Strong aromas may trigger nausea in people prone to it, and spices can irritate the mouth. The latter is of particular concern for people with mucositis, as spices may irritate mouth sores, causing severe discomfort.

In these instances, bland, cold food may be the most palatable.

General Dietary Guidelines for CLL Patients

For individuals managing chronic lymphocytic leukemia (CLL), maintaining a balanced diet is essential. Here are some tips to help:

Nourishing Foods: Focus on consuming foods rich in nutrients, especially if appetite is low.

Keep a Healthy Weight: It's important to maintain a healthy weight, so if unintentional weight loss occurs, consult with a healthcare provider.

Consider Supplements: Discuss with your healthcare team whether supplements could help ensure you're getting all the necessary nutrients.

Eat a Bit of Everything: Aim for a diet that includes a variety of fruits, vegetables, whole grains, lean proteins, and healthy fats.

Stay Hydrated: Drink plenty of fluids, particularly if treatments like chemotherapy lead to dehydration.

Follow the Rules: Adhere to any dietary guidelines provided by your healthcare team.

Tummy Troubles: Adjust your diet to ease gastrointestinal symptoms such as diarrhea or constipation.

Watch Your Bones: Ensure adequate intake of nutrients important for bone health, especially if undergoing treatments that may affect bone density.

Get Some Advice: Consider seeking guidance from a dietitian or nutrition expert familiar with CLL management.

Taking care of your diet can contribute to overall well-being while navigating CLL.

Foods to Include in a CLL Diet

Fruits and vegetables: Non-starchy vegetables and fruit, like broccoli, spinach, asparagus, bell peppers, apples, berries, and oranges, are nutritious and rich in fiber.

Grains: When choosing grain products, look for whole-grain foods. Processed grains have most of the vitamins and minerals stripped away. In addition, these foods usually contain more calories and sugar that are more likely to spike blood sugar. Focus on whole grain wheat products, oats, quinoa, and other unprocessed grains.

Protein: Try to choose leaner protein foods like poultry, fatty fish, eggs, and leaner cuts of red meat. Protein supports the growth of muscle and other body functions, helping to keep you healthy during cancer treatment. In addition, try to eat plant-based protein foods like beans, legumes, and nuts.

Foods to Limit or Avoid to Manage Symptoms and Treatment Side Effects

Desserts and processed foods: Sugary foods are associated with many chronic diseases and illnesses like cancer. Try to limit the number of times you eat dessert and processed foods.

Beverages: Aim for unsweetened drinks, like water, unsweetened tea, and coffee. Try to limit consumption of juice, soda, and other sweetened drinks.

Red Meat: While lean protein is important, it's advised to limit consumption of red meat. Opt for alternatives like chicken, turkey, or fish more frequently.

Sugar Intake: Limit sugary beverages, sweets, and desserts, as high sugar intake can affect immune function and promote inflammation. Choose whole fruits for sweetness instead.

Alcohol: If you choose to drink, do so in moderation as alcohol can weaken the immune system and may interfere with CLL medications.

Salt: Reduce consumption of salty snacks, canned soups, and processed foods. Instead, season meals with herbs and spices for flavor.

Raw or Undercooked Foods: Avoid foods like raw meats, seafood, eggs, and unpasteurized dairy products that may harbor harmful bacteria.

High-Fat Foods: Limit intake of fried foods, fatty meats, and full-fat dairy products as excessive saturated and trans fats can contribute to health issues.

Supplements: Consult with your healthcare provider before taking any supplements to ensure they are safe and won't interact with medications.

CHAPTER V: SAVORY RECIPES AND MEAL IDEAS FOR CLL DIET

SAVORY RECIPES AND MEAL IDEAS FOR BREAKFAST

Easy protein pancakes

Ingredients

1 banana

75g oats

3 large eggs

2 tbsp milk (dairy, soya, oat or nut milks all work)

1 tbsp baking powder

pinch of cinnamon

2 tbsp protein powder (whey, pea or whatever your preference)

coconut oil, or a flavourless oil, for frying

nut butter, maple syrup and berries or sliced banana to serve

Directions

STEP 1

Whizz the banana, oats, eggs, milk, baking powder, cinnamon and protein powder in a blender for 1-2 mins until smooth. Check the oats have broken down, if not, blend for another minute.

STEP 2

Heat a drizzle of oil in a pan. Pour or ladle in 2-3 rounds of batter, leaving a little space between each to spread. Cook for 1-2 minutes, until bubbles start to appear on the surface and the underside is golden. Flip over and cook for another minute until cooked through. Transfer to a warmed oven and repeat with the remaining batter. Serve in stacks with nut butter, maple syrup and fruit.

Berry omelette

Ingredients

1 large egg

1 tbsp skimmed milk

3 pinches of cinnamon

½ tsp rapeseed oil

100g cottage cheese

175g chopped strawberry, blueberries and raspberries

Directions

STEP 1

Beat egg with milk and cinnamon. Heat oil in a 20cm non-stick frying pan and pour in the egg mixture, swirling to evenly cover the base. Cook for a few mins until set and golden underneath. There's no need to flip it over.

STEP 2

Place on a plate, spread over cheese, then scatter with berries. Roll up and serve.

Cloud eggs

Ingredients

2 large eggs

2 tbsp chives, chopped

2 spring onions, finely sliced

wholemeal toast or gluten-free alternative, to serve (optional)

Directions

STEP 1

Heat oven to 230C/210C fan/gas 8. Separate the egg whites from the yolks. Tip the whites into a large, clean mixing bowl and beat with an electric whisk until aerated and fluffy.

STEP 2

Gently fold through 1½ tbsp of the chives and the spring onion. Line a baking sheet with baking parchment, then pile on the egg whites in two mounds. Use the back of a spoon to make a dip in the centre of each one. Bake for 8-10 mins until set and turning light golden brown. Gently tip the egg yolk into the centre of the egg whites and return to the oven for a further 2-3 mins, or until the yolk has just set. Serve sprinkled with the remaining chives. Eat on toast, or just as they come.

Staffordshire oatcakes with mushrooms

Ingredients

For the oatcakes

85g porridge oats

85g plain wholemeal flour

½ tsp dried yeast

For the topping

4 tsp rapeseed oil, plus a little for frying

320g button mushrooms, sliced

4 tomatoes, each cut into 8 wedges

4 tbsp milled seeds with flax and chia

4 tbsp tahini

a few coriander sprigs, chopped

Directions

STEP 1

For the oatcakes, tip the oats and 350ml water into a bowl and blitz with a stick blender until smooth (alternatively you can use a food processor or liquidizer). Stir in the flour and yeast, cover and leave in the fridge overnight, or leave at room temperature for 2-3 hrs until bubbles appear.

STEP 2

Use kitchen paper to rub ½ tsp oil round a non-stick frying pan, then heat. Ladle in a quarter of the batter and swirl the pan to cover the base (the oatcakes should be a few millimeters thick, like a crêpe). Cook for 2 mins, then turn and cook for 2 mins more until golden. Make four oatcakes in the same way.

STEP 3

To make the topping for two oatcakes, heat 2 tsp oil in a non-stick pan, add 160g mushrooms and fry for 2-3 mins, stirring until softened. Stir in 2 tomatoes, then add 2 tbsp ground seeds and cook for 2 mins more. Reheat the oatcakes in a dry frying pan or the microwave if necessary, then spread each one with 1 tbsp tahini, the mushroom mixture and scatter with a little coriander before serving. On the second day, repeat step 3 with the remaining Ingredients.

Overnight oats with apricots & yogurt

Ingredients

For the oats

200g oats

50g chia seeds

1 tbsp vanilla extract

550ml almond milk, or cow's milk (if non-vegan)

For the apricots

1 tsp rapeseed oil

320g pack fresh apricots, stoned and quartered

400g pot fortified oat or plain bio yogurt

4 tsp sunflower seeds

Directions

STEP 1

Mix the oats and chia in a bowl with the vanilla and almond milk. Cover and chill overnight.

STEP 2

Heat the oil in a small non-stick pan. Add the apricots in a single layer, then cover the pan and cook over a low heat for 5 mins, until softened. Stir well and cook a few minutes more if needed – they will cook a little more in the residual heat as they cool. Cover and keep chilled until needed.

STEP 3

The next day, stir the yogurt into the oats and spoon
into tumblers, small jars or small bowls. Top with the
cooked apricots and sunflower seeds. Will keep
covered and chilled for up to four days.

Warming chocolate & banana porridge

Ingredients

120g rolled porridge oats

4 tsp cocoa powder

1 tsp vanilla extract

4 bananas, 2 chopped

2 x 150ml pots bio yogurt

milk, to serve (optional)

Directions

STEP 1

Put the oats, cocoa and vanilla in a large bowl and pour over 800ml – 1 litre cold water (depending how thick you like your porridge). Cover the bowl and leave to soak overnight.

STEP 2

The next morning, tip the contents into a saucepan with the chopped banana. Cook over a medium heat for 15 mins, stirring frequently, until the oats are cooked.

STEP 3

Put half of the mixture in the fridge for the next day. Spoon the rest into two bowls, swirl in 1 pot yogurt and slice over a banana (save the other pot and banana for the next morning). Warm through with a splash of milk to reheat.

Butternut & cinnamon oats

Ingredients

120g porridge oats

80g raisins

2 tsp ground cinnamon, plus a sprinkling to serve

large chunk butternut squash, peeled and coarsely grated (approx 320g grated weight)

2 x 150ml pots bio yogurt

25g walnuts roughly broken

milk, to serve (optional)

Directions

STEP 1

Tip the oats, raisins and cinnamon into a large bowl and pour over 1 litre cold water. Cover the bowl and leave to soak overnight.

STEP 2

The next morning, tip the contents into a large saucepan and stir in the grated squash. Cook for about 8-10 mins over a medium heat, stirring frequently, until the oats are cooked and the squash is soft. Add a little more water if it's too thick.

STEP 3

Put half of the mixture in the fridge for the next day.

Spoon the remainder into bowls, top each portion with

1 pot yogurt and half the nuts. Dust with cinnamon,

then serve with a splash of milk.

Orange & raspberry granola

Ingredients

400g jumbo oats

juice 2 oranges (150ml), plus zest of 1/2

1 tsp ground cinnamon

2 tbsp freeze-dried raspberries or strawberries (see tip)

25g flaked almonds, toasted

25g mixed seeds (such as sunflower, pumpkin, sesame and linseed)

To serve

2 large oranges, peeled and segmented

mint leaves (optional)

Directions

STEP 1

Put 200g oats and 500ml water in a food processor and blitz for 1 min. Line a sieve with clean muslin and pour in the oat mixture. Leave to drip through for 5 mins, then twist the ends of the muslin and squeeze well to capture as much of the oat milk as possible – it should be the consistency of single cream. Best chilled at least 1 hr before serving. Can be kept in a sealed or covered jug in the fridge for up to 3 days.

STEP 2

Heat oven to 200C/180C fan/gas 6 and line a baking tray with baking parchment. Put the orange juice in a medium saucepan and bring to the boil. Boil rapidly for 5 mins or until the liquid has reduced by half, stirring occasionally. Mix the remaining 200g oats with the orange zest and cinnamon. Remove the pan from the heat and stir the oat mixture into the juice. Spread over the lined tray in a thin layer and bake for 10-15 mins or until lightly browned and crisp, turning the oats every few mins. Leave to cool on the tray.

STEP 3

Once cool, mix the oats with the raspberries, flaked almonds and seeds. Can be kept in a sealed jar for up to one week. To serve, spoon the granola into bowls, pour over the oat milk and top with the orange segments and mint leaves, if you like.

Scrambled egg muffin

Ingredients

2 eggs

few sundried tomatoes

fresh basil, torn

English muffins

Directions

STEP 1

Scramble eggs without butter or cream, stir in chopped sundried tomato and torn fresh basil, and pile on toasted English muffin halves.

Banana & cinnamon pancakes with blueberry compote

Ingredients

65g wholemeal flour

1 tsp ground cinnamon, plus extra for sprinkling

2 egg, plus 2 egg whites

100ml whole milk

1 small banana, mashed

½ tbsp rapeseed oil

320g blueberries

few mint leaves, to serve

Directions

STEP 1

Tip the flour and cinnamon into a bowl, then break in the whole eggs, pour in the milk and whisk together until smooth. Stir in the banana. In a separate bowl, whisk the egg whites until light and fluffy, but not completely stiff, then fold into the pancake mix until evenly incorporated.

STEP 2

Heat a small amount of oil in a large non-stick frying pan, then add a quarter of the pancake mix, swirl to cover the base of the pan and cook until set and golden. Carefully turn the pancake over with a palette knife and cook the other side. Transfer to a plate, then carry on with the rest of the batter until you have four.

STEP 3

To make the compote, tip the berries in a non-stick pan and heat gently until the berries just burst but hold their shape. Serve two warm pancakes with half the berries, then scatter with the mint leaves and sprinkle with a little cinnamon. Chill the remaining pancakes and compote and serve the next day. You can reheat them in the microwave or in a pan.

Pink barley porridge with vanilla yogurt

Ingredients

100g pearl barley

75g traditional oats

4 large or 8 small ripe red plums, stoned and chopped

½ tsp vanilla extract

4 x bio yogurt

2 tbsp sunflower seeds

Directions

STEP 1

Tip the barley and oats into a bowl, pour over 1 litre boiling water and stir well. Cover and leave to soak overnight.

STEP 2

The next morning, tip the mixture into a pan and stir in the plums. Simmer for 15 mins, stirring frequently and adding a little water if necessary to get a consistency you like.

STEP 3

Stir the vanilla into the yogurt and serve on top of the porridge with the seeds sprinkled over.

Winter fruit salad

Ingredients

600g good-quality ready-to-eat dried fruit (such as prunes, pears, apricots, figs cranberries)

3 tbsp clear honey

1 vanilla pod, split lengthways

1 Earl Grey tea bag

1 tbsp fresh lemon juice

mascarpone or Greek yogurt, to serve

Directions

STEP 1

Tip the fruits and 700ml/11⁄4 pints cold water into a large saucepan. Add the honey and vanilla, scraping the seeds from the pod into the pan. Bring to the boil. Stir well, lower the heat and simmer for 10 minutes until slightly syrupy.

STEP 2

Take the pan off the heat and stir in the tea bag. Leave to infuse for 10 minutes.

STEP 3

Discard the tea bag and vanilla pod, tip the fruits and liquid into a non-metallic bowl and pour over the lemon juice. Stir, then leave to cool. Cover and chill until ready to serve.

Malted walnut seed loaf

Ingredients

500g strong wholemeal flour (we used Doves Farm mixed grain malthouse bread flour)

7g sachet fast-action dried yeast

1 tsp salt

up to 350ml warm water

100g mixed seed (we used a mix of linseeds, hemp seeds, pumpkin seeds and sesame seeds)

50g walnut pieces

a little sunflower oil, for greasing

Directions

STEP 1

Make the dough with the flour, yeast, salt and water adding most of the seeds and all the walnuts as you knead the dough. Leave to rise in a clean bowl as stated, then knock back and shape into a large round. Roll the round in the remaining seeds, then lift the bread onto a tray to prove for about 30 mins until doubled in size.

STEP 2

Heat oven to 220C/fan 200C/gas 7. Bake the bread for 15 mins, then reduce the heat to 190C/fan 170C/gas 5 and continue to bake for 30 mins until the loaf sounds hollow when tapped on the base. Leave the bread on a cooling rack to cool completely. The loaf will stay fresh in an airtight container for 3 days or can be frozen for 1 month

SAVORY RECIPES AND MEAL IDEAS FOR LUNCH

Silvana's Mediterranean & basil pasta

Ingredients

2 red peppers, seeded and cut into chunks

2 red onions, cut into wedges

2 mild red chillies, seeded and diced

3 garlic cloves, coarsley chopped

1 tsp golden caster sugar

2 tbsp olive oil, plus extra to serve

1kg small ripe tomatoes, quartered

350g dried pasta

a handful of fresh basil leaves and 2 tbsp grated parmesan (or vegetarian alternative), to serve

Directions

STEP 1

To roast the veg, preheat the oven to 200C/gas 6/fan 180C. Scatter the peppers, red onions, chillies and garlic in a large roasting tin. Sprinkle with sugar, drizzle over the oil and season well with salt and pepper. Roast for 15 minutes, toss in the tomatoes and roast for another 15 minutes until everything is starting to soften and look golden.

STEP 2

While the vegetables are roasting, cook the pasta in a large pan of salted boiling water according to packet instructions, until tender but still with a bit of bite. Drain well.

STEP 3

Remove the vegetables from the oven, tip in the pasta and toss lightly together. Tear the basil leaves on top and sprinkle with Parmesan to serve. If you have any leftovers it makes a great cold pasta salad – just moisten with extra olive oil if needed.

Vegan chickpea curry jacket potatoes

Ingredients

4 sweet potatoes

1 tbsp coconut oil

1 ½ tsp cumin seeds

1 large onion, diced

2 garlic cloves, crushed

thumb-sized piece ginger, finely grated

1 green chilli, finely chopped

1 tsp garam masala

1 tsp ground coriander

½ tsp turmeric

2 tbsp tikka masala paste

2 x 400g can chopped tomatoes

2 x 400g can chickpeas, drained

lemon wedges and coriander leaves, to serve

Directions

STEP 1

Heat oven to 200C/180C fan/gas 6. Prick the sweet potatoes all over with a fork, then put on a baking tray and roast in the oven for 45 mins or until tender when pierced with a knife.

STEP 2

Meanwhile, melt the coconut oil in a large saucepan over medium heat. Add the cumin seeds and fry for 1 min until fragrant, then add the onion and fry for 7-10 mins until softened.

STEP 3

Put the garlic, ginger and green chilli into the pan, and cook for 2-3 mins. Add the spices and tikka masala paste and cook for a further 2 mins until fragrant, then tip in the tomatoes. Bring to a simmer, then tip in the chickpeas and cook for a further 20 mins until thickened. Season.

STEP 4

Put the roasted sweet potatoes on four plates and cut open lengthways. Spoon over the chickpea curry and squeeze over the lemon wedges. Season, then scatter with coriander before serving.

Herby fish fingers with Chinese-style rice

Ingredients

100g brown basmati rice

160g frozen peas

50g French beans

3 spring onions, finely chopped

½ tsp dried chilli flakes

good handful coriander, roughly chopped

2 tsp tamari

few drops sesame oil

1 tbsp cold-pressed rapeseed oil

2 large eggs

280g pack skinless cod loins cut into chunky strips (cut into 4 strips per loin)

Directions

STEP 1

Cook the rice in a pan of water for 25 mins, adding the peas and beans for the last 6 mins. Drain, then return to the pan and stir in the spring onions, chilli flakes, all but 1 tbsp chopped coriander, the tamari and sesame oil. Cover.

STEP 2

Meanwhile, heat a large non-stick pan with the rapeseed oil Beat the eggs with the remaining 1 tbsp coriander. Cut the fish into chunky strips, then coat them in the egg and fry in the oil for a couple of mins each side until golden. Remove the fish from the pan and tip in the rice with any remaining egg and stir. Serve in bowls, topped with the fish.

Rhubarb & date chutney

Ingredients

50g fresh root ginger, grated

300ml red wine vinegar

500g eating apple, peeled and finely chopped

200g pitted date, chopped

200g dried cranberries or raisins

1 tbsp mustard seed

1 tbsp curry powder

400g light muscovado sugar

700g rhubarb, sliced into 2cm chunks

500g red onion

Directions

STEP 1

Put the onions in a large pan with the ginger and vinegar. Bring to the boil, then simmer for 10 mins. Add the rest of the Ingredients, except the rhubarb, plus 2 tsp salt to the pan and bring to the boil, stirring. Simmer, uncovered, for about 10 mins until the apples are tender.

STEP 2

Stir in the rhubarb and cook, uncovered, until the chutney is thick and jammy, about 15-20 mins. Leave the chutney to sit for about 10-15 mins, then spoon into

warm, clean jars, and seal. Label the jars when cool.
Keep for at least a month before eating.

Herby broccoli & pea soup

Ingredients

1 tbsp rapeseed oil

1 onion, finely chopped

1 large garlic clove, crushed

400g broccoli, chopped into small florets

300g frozen peas

200g chard, chopped

1l low-salt veg stock

½ small bunch of basil, chopped

small bunch of dill, chopped

1 lemon, zested and juiced

2 tbsp pumpkin seeds, toasted

Directions

STEP 1

Heat the oil in a large saucepan. Add the onion and fry for 8 mins until soft and translucent. Add the garlic and cook for 1 min more. Tip in the broccoli, peas and chard, then pour over the stock and bring the mixture to the boil. Reduce the heat to a simmer, cover and cook for 25 mins.

STEP 2

Stir through the herbs, lemon zest and juice, then blitz the soup with a stick blender until completely smooth. Ladle into bowls and serve with the toasted pumpkin seeds scattered over the top.

Spinach kedgeree with spiced salmon

Ingredients

2 tsp rapeseed oil

1 large onion, halved and sliced

thumb-sized piece of ginger, finely chopped

½ tsp cumin seeds

½ tsp ground cinnamon

6-8 cardamom pods, seeds crushed

1½ tsp ground turmeric

1½ tsp ground coriander

1 red chilli, deseeded and sliced

1 garlic clove, finely chopped

1 large red pepper, deseeded and roughly chopped

70g brown basmati rice

375ml vegetable stock, made with 2 tsp bouillon powder

160g baby spinach leaves, roughly chopped

For the salmon

3 tbsp fat-free natural yogurt

1 tbsp finely chopped mint or coriander

2 skinless wild salmon fillets

1 tbsp toasted almonds, to serve

Directions

STEP 1

Heat the oil in a large frying pan and fry the onion and ginger for 5 mins or until soft. Add the cumin, cinnamon, crushed cardamom seeds, and 1 tsp each of the turmeric and coriander. Cook for 30 secs until fragrant. Add the chilli, garlic, pepper and rice, stir briefly, then pour in the stock. Cover and simmer for

35 mins or until the rice is tender and the stock has been absorbed. If the rice is cooked but some liquid remains, remove the lid and simmer uncovered to allow the liquid to evaporate. Add the spinach, cover and cook for 3 mins to wilt.

STEP 2

Meanwhile, prepare the salmon. Heat the grill to medium and line a baking sheet with foil. Mix the yogurt with the mint or coriander and the remaining turmeric and ground coriander. Spread the yogurt mixture over the salmon, then transfer to the prepared baking sheet and grill for 8-10 mins until the fish can be flaked easily with a fork. Top the kedgeree with the salmon fillets or flake the fish into it, and scatter over

the almonds to serve.

Pulled chicken salad

Ingredients

1 small roasted chicken, about 1kg

½ red cabbage, cored and finely sliced

3 carrots, coarsley grated or finely shredded

5 spring onions, finely sliced on the diagonal

2 red chillies, halved and thinly sliced

small bunch coriander, roughly chopped, including stalks

2 heaped tbsp roasted salted peanuts, roughly crushed

For the dressing

3 ½ tbsp hoisin sauce

1 ½ tbsp toasted sesame oil

Directions

STEP 1

Combine the dressing Ingredients in a small bowl and
set aside.

STEP 2

Remove all the meat from the chicken, shred into large
chunks and pop in a large bowl. Add the cabbage,
carrots, spring onions, chillies and half the coriander.
Toss together with the dressing and pile onto a serving
plate, then scatter over the remaining coriander and
peanuts.

Air fryer baked potatoes

Ingredients

4 baking potatoes (about 250g each)

½ tbsp sunflower oil

toppings of your choice, such as butter, cheese, baked beans or tuna mayonnaise

Directions

STEP 1

Scrub the potatoes, then pat dry with kitchen paper. Transfer to a plate, drizzle over the oil and rub it into the skins using your hands so the potatoes are well-coated. Season with salt and pepper – the salt will help the skins crisp up.

STEP 2

Arrange the potatoes in a single layer in an air fryer basket. Set the air fryer to 200C and cook for 40-50 mins, or until a sharp knife goes through the potatoes easily. Check the potatoes after 20 mins – if they seem to be browning too quickly on one side, turn them over using tongs, then check again after another 20 mins to ensure they're cooked through. The size of the potato and model of airfryer may effect the cooking time. To speed up the cooking time, you can microwave on high for 8-10 mins before airfrying (check after 15-20 mins). When ready, the skin should be crisp and the inside tender and fluffy. Split and serve immediately with the toppings of your choice.

Ginger chicken & green bean noodles

Ingredients

½ tbsp vegetable oil

2 skinless chicken breasts, sliced

200g green beans, trimmed and halved crosswise

thumb-sized piece of ginger, peeled and cut into matchsticks

2 garlic cloves, sliced

1 ball stem ginger, finely sliced, plus 1 tsp syrup from the jar

1 tsp cornflour, mixed with 1 tbsp water

1 tsp dark soy sauce, plus extra to serve (optional)

2 tsp rice vinegar

200g cooked egg noodles

Directions

STEP 1

Heat the oil in a wok over a high heat and stir-fry the chicken for 5 mins. Add the green beans and stir-fry for 4-5 mins more until the green beans are just tender, and the chicken is just cooked through.

STEP 2

Stir in the fresh ginger and garlic, and stir-fry for 2 mins, then add the stem ginger and syrup, the cornflour mix, soy sauce and vinegar. Stir-fry for 1 min, then toss in the noodles. Cook until everything is hot and the sauce coats the noodles. Drizzle with more soy, if you like, and serve.

Feta & kale loaded sweet potato

Ingredients

2 sweet potatoes

chickpeas, drained

1 red onion, thinly sliced

2tbsp red wine vinegar

30g feta, cut into small cubes

1 tsp caster sugar

1tbsp olive oil

chilli flakes

100g kale

1tbsp pumpkin seeds, toasted

rocket

Directions

STEP 1

Heat oven to 200C/180C fan/gas 6. Prick the sweet potatoes all over with a fork, then put them in a roasting tin and roast for 40 mins. Add the chickpeas to the tray, then roast for 10 mins more, until the potatoes are completely tender and the chickpeas have crisped a little.

STEP 2

Meanwhile, mix the onion with the vinegar and a pinch of sugar and salt, and set aside to quick pickle. In another bowl, marinate the feta with the oil and chilli flakes.

STEP 3

When the potatoes are nearly cooked, cook the kale in a pan with 50ml water for 3 mins until wilted, then season to taste. Halve the potatoes, divide between two plates and top each with the kale, chickpeas, red onion (reserving the vinegar), marinated feta and pumpkin seeds. Toss the rocket with the reserved vinegar, then serve on the side.

Super-green mackerel salad

Ingredients

85g green bean

85g thin-stemmed broccoli

large handful baby spinach leaves

2 hot-smoked mackerel fillets (about 75g), skinned and flaked

2 tsp sunflower seed, toasted

For the dressing

75ml low-fat natural yogurt

1 tsp lemon juice

1 tsp wholegrain mustard

2 tsp dill, chopped, plus extra to serve

Directions

STEP 1

Boil a pan of water. Add the green beans and cook for 2 mins, then add the broccoli and cook for 4 mins more. Drain, run under cold water until cool, then drain well.

STEP 2

To make the dressing, combine all the Ingredients in a small jam jar with a twist of black pepper, put the lid on and give it a good shake.

STEP 3

To serve, mix together the cooked veg with the spinach and mackerel and pack into a lunchbox. Just before eating, pour over the dressing, scatter over the sunflower seeds and add a grind of black pepper and extra dill.

Spiced chickpea soup

Ingredients

1 tbsp olive oil

1 onion, chopped

2 garlic cloves, crushed

1 red chilli, deseeded and roughly chopped

1 tbsp grated fresh ginger

1 tsp cumin

1 tsp ras-el-hanout

¼ tsp cinnamon

200g roasted red pepper, from a jar

2 x 400g cans chopped tomato

400ml vegetable stock

400g can chickpea, drained and rinsed

2 preserved lemons, rind chopped (discard the pulp and seeds)

1 tbsp clear honey

50g wholewheat couscous

Directions

STEP 1

Heat the oil in a large lidded pan. Add the onion and garlic, put on the lid and cook for 5 mins, stirring halfway through. Stir the chilli, ginger, cumin, ras el hanout and cinnamon into the pan and cook for 1 min. Add the peppers, tomatoes and stock. Bring to the boil, turn down to a simmer, put on the lid and cook for 10 mins.

STEP 2

Blitz the soup with a stick blender, or in a food processor until smooth. Return to the pan and add more liquid to thin the soup, if you like. Stir in the chickpeas, preserved lemons, honey and some seasoning. If eating straight away, add the couscous and heat through for 5 mins. (If taking to work, add the couscous just before reheating).

Cullen skink

Ingredients

1 tbsp unsalted butter

1 medium onion

400g medium potatoes (about 2), peeled and cut into 1cm cubes

250g smoked haddock

250ml whole milk

½ small bunch of parsley or chives, finely chopped

Directions

STEP 1

Melt the butter in a saucepan over a medium heat, then add the onion and fry for 5-8 mins until translucent but not browned. Add the potatoes and 300ml water and bring to the boil. Reduce the heat slightly and simmer for 10-15 mins.

STEP 2

Meanwhile, put the haddock in another pan and cover with the the milk. Cook gently for 5 mins, or until just tender. Remove the haddock from the milk with a slotted spoon (reserving the milk), transfer to a plate and leave to cool slightly. When cool enough to touch, flake into large pieces, removing any bones.

STEP 3

Put the reserved milk and flaked haddock in the pan with the potato mixture and cook for another 5 mins. Season and sprinkle over the parsley to serve.

Chicken tacos

Ingredients

250g plain flour, plus extra for dusting

2 tbsp rapeseed oil

2 tbsp taco or fajita seasoning (see tip, below)

5-6 skinless chicken breasts, sliced

¼ red cabbage, finely shredded

3 limes, 1 juiced, 2 cut into wedges

small bunch of coriander, chopped

4 sweetcorn cob, kernels sliced off, or 400g frozen sweetcorn

400g can black beans, drained and rinsed

2 garlic cloves, crushed

4 tbsp fat-free yogurt, to serve

chilli sauce, to serve

Directions

STEP 1

Combine the flour with half the oil and a small pinch of salt in a bowl. Pour over 125-150ml warm water, then bring together into a soft dough with your hands. Cut into six equal pieces, then cut four of the pieces in half again, so you have eight small pieces and two large. Roll all the pieces out on a floured work surface until they're as thin as you can get them.

STEP 2

Heat a dry frying pan over a medium-high heat and cook the small and large tortillas for 2-3 mins on each side until golden and toasted (do this one at a time). Leave the large tortillas to cool, then cover and reserve for use in the lunchboxes (see tip below). Keep the small tortillas warm in foil.

STEP 3

Sprinkle the taco seasoning over the chicken in a bowl, and toss to combine. Toss the cabbage with the lime juice, half the coriander and some seasoning in another bowl, then leave to pickle.

STEP 4

Meanwhile, heat two frying pans over a high heat. Divide the remaining oil between the pans and fry the sweetcorn and a pinch of salt until sizzling and turning golden, stirring occasionally – you want the sweetcorn to char slightly, as this adds flavour, so you may need to leave it to cook undisturbed for a bit. While the sweetcorn cooks and chars, fry the chicken in the larger pan until cooked through and golden (you may need to do this in batches).

STEP 5

Tip the black beans and garlic into the sweetcorn and stir to warm through. Squeeze over two of the lime wedges.

STEP 6

Reserve two spoonfuls each of the chicken (about 1 chicken breast) and sweetcorn mix for use in the lunchboxes (see tip, below), then serve the rest in bowls alongside the cabbage, yogurt, lime wedges, remaining coriander, chilli sauce and tortillas for everyone to dig into.

SAVORY RECIPES AND MEAL IDEAS FOR DINNER

Faggots with onion gravy

Ingredients

little oil, for the tin

170g pack sage & onion stuffing mix (we used Paxo)

500g pack diced pork shoulder

300g pig liver

½ tsp ground mace

For the gravy

2 onions, thinly sliced

1 tbsp sunflower oil

2 tsp sugar

1 tbsp red wine vinegar

3 tbsp plain flour

850ml beef stock

handful chopped parsley

mash and veg, to serve (optional)

Directions

STEP 1

Heat oven to 160C/140C fan/gas 3. Lightly oil a very large roasting tin. Tip the stuffing mix into a large bowl, add 500ml boiling water, stir and set aside.

STEP 2

Pulse the pork in a food processor until finely chopped. Add the liver and pulse again. Add to the stuffing with the mace, 1 tsp salt and plenty of black pepper. Stir well. Shape the mixture (it will be very soft) into 24 large faggots and put in the prepared tin.

STEP 3

To make the gravy, fry the onions in the oil until starting to turn golden. Add the sugar and continue cooking, stirring frequently, until caramelised. Tip in the vinegar and allow to sizzle. Mix the flour with a couple of tbsp water. Pour the stock into the onions, then add the flour paste and cook, stirring constantly, until smooth and starting to thicken. When it is thick, pour into the tin with the faggots, cover with foil and bake for 1 hr until cooked through. Serve sprinkled with parsley, with mash and a veg, if you like.

Squid, prawn & chickpea nduja stew

Ingredients

2 tbsp olive oil

1 onion, finely chopped

1 fennel, finely chopped, fronds reserved

2 garlic cloves, sliced

1 tbsp nduja or 1 cooking chorizo, skin removed, crumbled

400g can chopped tomatoes

100ml red wine

250ml chicken stock

400g can chickpeas, drained

200g prepared squid

200g king prawns (peeled weight)

small handful of flat-leaf parsley, chopped

1 lemon, zested

Directions

STEP 1

Heat the olive oil in a large, flameproof shallow casserole dish over a medium heat, and cook the onion, fennel and garlic for 12 mins, stirring occasionally until soft and just turning golden. Stir in the nduja or chorizo and sizzle for 2 mins until the oils are released and the veg starts to take on the red colour.

STEP 2

Tip in the tomatoes, then rinse the can out with the wine and pour it in, along with the stock. Stir in the chickpeas. Season and bring to a simmer, then cook for 20 mins until the sauce is rich. Season to taste.

STEP 3

Stir in the squid and prawns so they're completely mixed into the sauce, then simmer for about 5 mins more until the squid and prawns are cooked through. Scatter with the parsley, lemon zest and reserved fennel fronds before serving.

Cod with olives & crispy pancetta

Ingredients

100g pack olives & sundried tomatoes

2tbsp olive oil

400g can chopped tomatoes

4 skinless cod fillets

8 slices thin pancetta

Directions

STEP 1

Mix the olives & sundried tomatoes with the chopped

tomatoes, then season. Tip the sauce into a casserole

dish, top with the fish and drizzle over 2 tbsp olive oil.
Bake at 200C/180C fan/gas 6 for 15-20 mins or until the
fish is just cooked. Heat a medium frying pan until hot,
add the pancetta and cook on both sides for 1 min or
until crisp. Top the fish with shards of the pancetta.

Fresh salmon with Thai noodle salad

Ingredients

2 skinless salmon fillets

1 large orange, the juice and zest of half, the rest peeled
and chopped

125g French beans, trimmed and halved

50g mange tout, shredded

75g frozen peas

75g vermicelli rice noodles

2 tsp red curry paste

1 tsp fish sauce

3 spring onions, finely chopped

half a pack basil or coriander, chopped

Directions

STEP 1

Put a pan of water on to boil. Line a steamer with baking parchment, add the salmon fillets and scatter with a little of the orange zest. When the water is boiling, add the beans to the pan, put the salmon in the steamer on top and cook for 5 mins. Take the salmon off, and if it is cooked, set aside but add the peas and mange tout to the pan and cook for 1 min more, or if not quite cooked leave on top for the extra min. Drain the veg, but return the boiling water to the pan, add the noodles and leave to soak for 5 mins.

STEP 2

Put the curry paste and fish sauce in a salad bowl with the orange juice and a little of the remaining zest and the spring onions. Drain the noodles when they are ready and add to the salad bowl, toss well, then add the chopped orange with the basil or coriander and the cooked vegetables. Tip in the juice from the fish, then toss well and serve in bowls with the salmon on top.

Vegetarian moussaka

Ingredients

140g dried green lentils

2 onions, halved and sliced

2 garlic cloves, chopped

2 bay leaves

1 tsp dried oregano

½ tsp cinnamon

½tsp allspice

400g can chopped tomatoes

1 cube reduced-salt vegetable stock

200g sweet potato, thinly sliced

1 large aubergine, sliced and the biggest slices halved again

300g full-fat plain yogurt

60g plain flour

2 egg yolks

120g mature cheddar, finely grated

2-3 tomatoes, cut into slices (optional)

Directions

STEP 1

Heat the oven to 180C/160C fan/gas 4. Put the lentils, onions, garlic, herbs and spices in a large pan, and pour in 850ml water. Bring to the boil, cover and simmer for 10 mins.

STEP 2

Tip in the tomatoes, stock cube, sweet potato and aubergine, then cover and simmer for a further 20-25 mins until the lentils and veg are tender, and the liquid has been absorbed. Remove the bay leaves. Add salt and pepper to taste.

STEP 3

Place the yogurt, flour and egg yolks together in a bowl and whisk. Set aside. Spread the filling out in a large baking dish and cover with the topping evenly. Spread over the yogurt mixture, right to the edges. Sprinkle the cheddar over the top, then add the tomato slices, if using. Bake for 30-40 mins until the topping is golden and bubbling. Will keep for up to three days in the fridge.

Harissa fish with bulgur salad

Ingredients

100g bulgur wheat

½ small cucumber, deseeded and finely chopped

100g cherry tomatoes, quartered

25g pitted green olives

small handful of parsley, finely chopped

2tbsp rose harissa

2tsp honey

1 garlic clove, crushed

½ lemon, juiced

2tbsp olive oil

½ red onion, finely sliced

2 x 120g skinless, boneless white fish fillets, such as cod or haddock

Directions

STEP 1

Cook the bulgur following pack instructions, then rinse and drain well before tipping into a large bowl.

Add the cucumber, tomatoes, olives and most of the parsley. Season well. Combine the harissa, honey, garlic, lemon juice, half the oil and 1 tbsp water in a bowl, then set aside.

STEP 2

Heat the remaining oil in a non-stick pan over a medium heat and cook the red onion for 4-5 mins until softened and lightly browned. Season the fish well, then add to the pan and cook for 3 mins before pouring in the harissa mixture. Turn the fish and cook for 2-4 mins more (depending on the thickness of the fish), basting the fish in the pan juices until cooked through – the flesh should be opaque.

STEP 3

Divide the bulgur salad between two plates, top with the fish and fried onions, then drizzle over any remaining pan juices and sprinkle over the remaining parsley to serve.

Chicken sausage pasta

Ingredients

1 tbsp sunflower oil

1 onion, chopped

400g chicken sausage, sliced

1 large garlic clove, crushed or finely grated

200g roasted red peppers, chopped

1 tsp ground cumin (optional)

½ tsp chilli flakes (optional)

400g can chopped tomatoes

100g spinach

500g penne or rigatoni pasta

Directions

STEP 1

Heat the oil in a large lidded frying pan or saucepan
over a medium heat and fry the onion for 5 mins until
beginning to soften. Tip in the sausage pieces and fry

for 4-5 mins until beginning to brown. Tip in the garlic, peppers, cumin and chilli, if using, season well and stir to combine. Cook for 2-3 mins more until fragrant, then tip in the chopped tomatoes and half a can of water. Reduce the heat to a simmer and cook for another 10-15 mins until the liquid has reduced a little and the sausages are cooked through. Add the spinach, stir, cover and cook for 3-5 mins more until the spinach has wilted, then mix to combine.

STEP 2

Meanwhile, cook the pasta following pack instructions. Drain, reserving a cupful of the pasta water.

STEP 3

Tip the cooked pasta into the sauce and stir gently to combine. Cook for a 2-3 mins, then stir in some of the reserved pasta water if the sauce needs to be loosened. Serve.

Air-fryer tuna pasta bake

Ingredients

1 tbsp olive oil

1 small onion, finely chopped

2 garlic cloves, finely chopped

400g can chopped tomatoes

½ tsp chilli flakes (optional)

150g pasta of your choice, cooked following pack
instructions

145-165g can tuna in olive oil, drained

50g grated mozzarella

2 tbsp chopped parsley

Directions

STEP 1

Heat the air-fryer to 190C. Tip the oil, onion and garlic into a heatproof dish and air-fry for 3 mins. Add the tomatoes and chilli flakes, if using, along with some seasoning. Air-fry for a further 5 mins.

STEP 2

Reduce the temperature to 170C. Stir in the cooked pasta, tuna, most of the mozzarella and the parsley. Scatter the reserved mozzarella over the top.

STEP 3

Air-fry for 5 mins until golden, then cover with foil and cook for a further 5 mins until bubbling. Serve warm with salad.

Slow cooker turkey curry

Ingredients

1 onion, chopped

4 garlic cloves, crushed or finely grated

thumb-sized piece ginger, peeled and finely grated

1 red pepper, chopped

350g sweet potatoes peeled and roughly chopped (you can also use carrots, parsnips or other root veg)

700g turkey, cut into large pieces (or use the same amount of leftover roasted turkey)

400g can chickpeas, drained and rinsed

2 tbsp curry paste (we used balti)

1 tbsp tomato purée

400g can chopped tomatoes

400g can coconut milk

small bunch of coriander, leaves picked and stalks reserved, both finely chopped

120g spinach (optional)

cooked rice, to serve

Directions

STEP 1

Tip the onion, garlic, ginger, red pepper, sweet potatoes, turkey and chickpeas into a slow cooker. Stir in the curry paste and tomato purée, ensuring everything is well-coated. Pour in the chopped tomatoes and coconut milk, and scatter in the chopped coriander stalks, 1 tsp salt and some ground black pepper. Mix everything to combine. Cook on high for 3 hrs 30 mins, or low for 8 hrs. If you want to add spinach, tip it in 15 mins before the end of the cooking time. Stir well after 5 mins, once it has started to wilt.

STEP 2

Serve the turkey curry with rice, scattered with the chopped coriander leaves, if you like.

Turmeric chicken with butter bean hummus & roasted peppers

Ingredients

1 large red pepper, halved and deseeded

1 tsp vegetable oil

160g long-stem broccoli

handful of mint leaves, to serve

For the chicken and marinade

2 large skinless chicken breast fillets (about 125g each)

120g natural yogurt

3 tbsp finely grated turmeric

½ tsp cumin seeds

½ tsp ground coriander

1 garlic clove, finely grated

1 tbsp lemon juice

1 tsp honey

1 tsp extra virgin olive oil

For the butter bean hummus

400g can butter beans, drained, liquid reserved

1 tbsp lemon zest, plus 1 tbsp lemon juice

1 tbsp extra virgin olive oil, plus a drizzle

1 garlic clove, roughly chopped

½ tsp cumin seeds

½ tsp ground coriander

Directions

STEP 1

Heat the oven to 220C/200C fan/gas 7. Line a baking sheet with foil. Make a few small cuts around the edges of the pepper halves using a sharp knife, then flatten them as much as you can with your palm. Rub with the veg oil and roast on the lined baking sheet for 10 mins.

STEP 2

Meanwhile, cut the chicken breasts in half lengthways at an angle so you end up with four thin fillets. Mix the yogurt, turmeric, cumin seeds, ground coriander, garlic, lemon juice, honey and olive oil with some black pepper and 1 tsp salt in a bowl. Add the chicken and turn to coat in the marinade. When the peppers have had 10 mins, turn them over, add the chicken fillets to the sheet, spacing them apart slightly, and spoon any remaining marinade over them. Roast for 20 mins, turning the chicken fillets halfway, until cooked through.

STEP 3

For the hummus, use a hand blender to blitz together the beans, lemon zest and juice, olive oil, garlic, cumin seeds and coriander with 6 tbsp liquid from the can, ¾ tsp salt and plenty of black pepper. It should be completely smooth.

STEP 4

When the chicken has been cooking for 10 mins, steam the broccoli for 6 mins until tender. Spoon the hummus over two plates, then top with the roasted peppers and

chicken. Scatter with the mint, drizzle with olive oil

and serve with the broccoli on the side.

Beef stew & dumplings

Ingredients

For the stew

1 tbsp rapeseed oil

2 medium onions, chopped

2 bay leaves

4 thyme sprigs, plus extra leaves to serve

550g chunks of lean braising steak

100ml red wine

1 ½ tbsp plain flour

1 tsp English mustard powder

230g can plum tomatoes

500ml vegetable bouillon

280g carrots, halved lengthways and sliced

400g piece butternut squash, deseeded, peeled and cut
into 3-4cm/11/4-11/2in chunks

140g chestnut mushrooms, quartered or halved if large

For the dumplings

140g self-raising flour

½ tsp English mustard powder

2 spring onions, ends trimmed, finely chopped

3 tbsp chopped parsley

2 tbsp rapeseed oil

100ml buttermilk

Directions

STEP 1

Heat the oil in a large saucepan or deep sauté pan. Tip
in the onions, bay leaves and thyme sprigs, and fry
over a medium heat for about 8 mins, stirring often,
until the onions are turning golden. Raise the heat, add
the steak and stir-fry briefly until it starts to lose its
raw, red colour. Pour in the wine, stir to deglaze the
brown sticky bits from the bottom of the pan, and let it
bubble briefly. Lower the heat, sprinkle in the flour and
mustard powder, and stir for 1 min. The meat should
now be coated in a thick, rich sauce.

STEP 2

Mix in the tomatoes, stirring to break them down. Stir in the stock and bring to the boil. Tip in the carrots, squash and mushrooms, lower the heat, cover with a lid and leave to simmer gently for 1 hr 40 mins, stirring occasionally. Uncover and cook for a further 20 mins, still on a gentle simmer, until the meat is very tender. Season with pepper.

STEP 3

When the stew is nearly cooked, heat oven to 190C/170C fan/gas 5. Put a 2.25-litre casserole dish in to heat it up. Meanwhile, make the dumplings. Put the flour, mustard powder, some pepper and a pinch of salt in a bowl, then stir in the spring onions and parsley. Mix the oil and buttermilk together and gently stir into the flour. Add a drop or two of cold water, if needed, to pick up any dry bits on the bottom of the bowl, and stir to make a soft and slightly sticky dough. Be as light-handed as you can, as overmixing or overhandling will toughen the dumplings. Cut the dough into 8 pieces and very lightly shape each into a small, rough ball.

STEP 4

Carefully transfer the stew to the hot casserole dish and remove the bay leaves and thyme sprigs. Sit the dumplings on top and press them down into the gravy to very slightly submerge. Put the dish on a baking sheet and cook for about 20 mins until the dumplings have risen and are golden on top. Serve with a light scattering of thyme leaves.

Inside-out chicken kiev

Ingredients

4 skinless, boneless chicken breasts

25g garlic butter, softened

25g crispy breadcrumbs

Directions

STEP 1

Place the chicken on a baking tray, rub with a little of the butter, season and cook under the grill for 15 mins, turning once until cooked through.

STEP 2

Mix together the remaining garlic butter and breadcrumbs. Remove the chicken from the grill and top each breast with a smear of the breadcrumbed butter. Return to the grill and cook 3-5 mins until the breadcrumbs are golden and the butter melted. Serve any buttery juices, alongside new potatoes and peas or broad beans.

Chicken schnitzel with coleslaw

Ingredients

For the schnitzel

4 small chicken breasts

3 tbsp grated parmesan

100g flour

1 large egg, beaten

75g dried breadcrumbs (we used panko)

75ml vegetable oil

For the coleslaw

300g white cabbage, shredded

1 large carrot, peeled and grated

6 spring onions, sliced diagonally

1 red-skinned apple, grated

150g pot natural yogurt

juice ½ lemon

2 tsp English mustard

Directions

STEP 1

For the coleslaw, mix all the Ingredients in a large bowl. Season a little and set aside.

STEP 2

Place a layer of cling film on your work surface and pop the chicken fillets on top. Cover with another piece of cling film and, using a rolling pin, bash the chicken until it is 2-3mm thick.

STEP 3

Put the flour on a plate and season, then put the egg on another plate. Dip the chicken in the flour to coat, then into the egg.

STEP 4

Mix together the breadcrumbs and Parmesan in a shallow bowl, then toss the chicken in the mixture to completely coat in the crumbs. Put the chicken on a plate and chill in the fridge until ready to eat if you're not cooking them straight away.

STEP 5

Heat the oil in a large frying pan over a fairly high heat and cook the chicken schnitzels two at a time. Sizzle them for 2-3 mins each side until completely golden, then lift out onto kitchen paper to drain. You can keep them warm in a low oven while you cook the rest. Serve with the coleslaw.

SAVORY RECIPES AND MEAL IDEAS FOR SNACK

Bean & feta spread with Greek salad salsa & oatcakes

Ingredients

400g can butter beans, drained

1 lemon, ½ juiced, ½ cut into 4 wedges

2 tbsp ricotta or bio yogurt

85g feta, crumbled

1 garlic clove

12 oatcakes

For the salsa

4 tomatoes, chopped

1 medium cucumber, finely diced

1 small red onion, finely chopped

12 pitted Kalamata olives, chopped

a few chopped mint leaves (optional)

Directions

STEP 1

Tip the beans, lemon juice, ricotta, 50g feta and the garlic into a bowl and blitz with a hand blender or in a food processor to make a paste. Stir in the remaining feta and spoon the mixture into four small pots.

STEP 2

To make the salsa, stir all the Ingredients together with the mint (if using) and divide into four more pots, topping with a lemon wedge. These will keep, chilled in an airtight container, for two-three days. To eat, spread the oatcakes with the bean mixture, squeeze the lemon wedges over the salads and pile generously onto the oatcakes.

Smoky veggie nachos

Ingredients

7 soft corn tortillas

1 tbsp rapeseed oil

1 tsp sweet smoked paprika, plus extra to serve

2 red peppers, halved and deseeded

400g can black beans, drained and rinsed

½ bunch of parsley, very finely chopped

50g fat-free yogurt

1 jalapeño, finely sliced

For the salsa

4 spring onions, finely sliced

4 medium tomatoes, deseeded and finely chopped

1 small avocado, peeled, stoned and chopped

½ small bunch of coriander, finely chopped

1 small garlic clove, finely grated

1 lime, zested and juiced

1 tbsp rapeseed oil

Directions

STEP 1

Heat the oven to 180C/160C fan/ gas 4. Cut each of the tortillas into 8-10 triangles and spread over two large baking sheets. Drizzle with the oil and sprinkle over the paprika. Bake for 7-8 mins until crisp and leave to cool.

STEP 2

Heat the grill to high. Grill the peppers, skin-side up, for 7-10 mins until charred and soft. Leave to cool. Peel off and discard the skins, slice into strips and toss with the beans and parsley.

STEP 3

To make the salsa, combine the Ingredients. Pile the nachos on a large plate, top with the bean mix, salsa, yogurt and jalapeño and sprinkle over some paprika to serve.

Date & peanut butter dip

Ingredients

1 tbsp crunchy peanut butter (30g)

2 dates, finely chopped (10g)

120g bio yogurt

1-2 sticks celery, cut into shorter, thinner lengths

1 green pepper, deseeded and cut into strips

Directions

STEP 1

Mash the peanut butter and dates together using a fork, then stir in the yogurt. Divide between two small bowls, or pots with lids for packing into lunchboxes. Will keep covered and chilled for up to three days. Serve with the vegetables for dipping.

Mozzarella, pepper & aubergine calzone

Ingredients

400g strong wholewheat bread flour, plus extra for dusting

⅛ tsp salt (optional)

7g sachet fast-action dried yeast

2 tsp rapeseed oil, plus extra for the baking sheet

For the filling

2 tsp rapeseed oil

1 red and 1 yellow pepper, deseeded and cut into small chunks

1 large aubergine, halved lengthways and thinly sliced

2 large garlic cloves, finely chopped

1 tbsp tomato purée

1 tbsp balsamic vinegar

small bunch basil, roughly torn

8 pitted Kalamata olives, halved

125g ball mozzarella (drained weight), quartered

milk or beaten egg, for brushing

Directions

STEP 1

Put the flour, salt (if using), yeast, oil and 300ml lukewarm water in a bowl and mix until soft. Knead into a ball (try not to add any extra flour) – it will be sticky but the flour will absorb some moisture. Return to the bowl, cover and leave somewhere warm.

STEP 2

Meanwhile, make the filling. Heat the oil in a large non-stick pan, then stir-fry the peppers for about 1 min until they start to soften. Add the aubergine and garlic and continue to cook over a medium heat for 8-10 mins, gently pressing the veg with a wooden spoon until it breaks down a little. If it doesn't, fry, covered, for a few extra mins.

STEP 3

Stir in the tomato purée, vinegar and 2 tbsp water. When the veg is soft, remove the pan from the heat and stir through the basil.

STEP 4

Heat the oven to 220C/200C fan/gas 7. Quarter the risen dough and roll each piece out to a 20cm circle on a lightly floured surface. Spoon a quarter of the filling over one side, scatter over a quarter of the olives, top with a quarter of the cheese, and brush the edges with the milk or beaten egg. Fold the dough over the filling and pinch the edges together at the side, a bit like making a Cornish pasty. Lift onto a lightly oiled baking sheet and brush with more milk or beaten egg. Repeat with the remaining dough and filling to make four calzones, then bake for 15-20 mins until golden. Leave to cool slightly and serve at room temperature.

Chicken skewers with tzatziki

Ingredients

2 tsp oregano

1 garlic clove

1 small yellow pepper

1 small red pepper

wholemeal tortilla wraps, to serve

baby spinach leaves, to serve

few sprigs flat-leaf parsley, to serve

For the tzatziki

½ cucumber

¼ garlic clove

4 tbsp Greek yogurt

1 tbsp extra virgin olive oil

You will need

eight bamboo skewers

Directions

STEP 1

Soak eight bamboo skewers in water. Using sharp kitchen scissors, chop the chicken into small pieces. Pop into a plastic box with a lid. Pare strips of lemon zest from the lemon using a vegetable peeler, then juice the lemon as well. Add both the peel and the juice to the chicken in the box along with the oregano and the garlic, crushed in. Season generously, mix and put in the fridge for 15 mins with the lid on. Deseed and chop the peppers into similar-sized pieces to those of the chicken.

STEP 2

Heat a griddle pan to high while you get the chicken out. Discard the lemon zest and thread the chicken onto the skewers, alternating every few bits of chicken with a piece of red pepper followed by a piece of yellow pepper. Griddle for 10 mins, turning halfway.

STEP 3

While the skewers are cooking, make the tzatziki. Get a box grater and a bowl. Cut the cucumber into long lengths, discarding the watery seedy core. Grate into the bowl, then grate the ¼ garlic clove. Season generously and stir in the Greek yogurt. Drizzle with a little extra virgin olive oil.

STEP 4

Serve the skewers hot off the griddle with the dip, or take the chicken and peppers off the skewers, leave to cool and pack into wholemeal wraps spread with a little tzatziki and rolled up with baby spinach and a few picked leaves of parsley.

Carrot & hummus roll-ups

Ingredients

200g tub hummus

4 seeded wraps

4 carrots

small handful rocket leaves

Directions

STEP 1

Spread the hummus between wraps. Coarsely grate carrots and scatter on top of the hummus, finishing each wrap with a small handful of rocket leaves and some seasoning. Roll up and eat.

Peanut hummus with fruit & veg sticks

Ingredients

380g carton chickpeas

zest and juice 0.5 lemon (use the other 1/2 to squeeze over the apple to stop it browning, if you like)

1 tbsp tahini

0.5-1 tsp smoked paprika

2 tbsp roasted unsalted peanuts

1 tsp rapeseed oil

2 crisp red apples, cored and cut into slices

2 carrots, cut into sticks

4 celery sticks, cut into batons lengthways

Directions

STEP 1

Drain the chickpeas, reserving the liquid. Tip three-quarters of the chickpeas into a food processor and add the lemon zest and juice, tahini, paprika, peanuts and oil with 3 tbsp chickpea liquid. Blitz in a food processor until smooth, then stir in the reserved chickpeas. Serve with the fruit and veg sticks.

Pumpkin hummus

Ingredients

1 small pumpkin (about 500g)

olive oil, for roasting

2 garlic cloves, peeled

½ lemon, juiced

2 tbsp tahini paste

400g can chickpeas, drained

1 red pepper, deseeded, and sliced

1 yellow pepper, deseeded, and sliced

mini breadsticks and pitta chips, to serve

Directions

STEP 1

Cut the top off the pumpkin, about two-thirds of the way up. Remove the pumpkin seeds, then scoop the flesh out of the bottom and the lid.

STEP 2

Heat oven to 200C/180C fan/gas 6. Cut the pumpkin flesh into pieces and put in a roasting tin with the garlic and a good glug of oil. Season, then bake for 45 mins until very tender. Leave to cool.

STEP 3

Tip the pumpkin into a food processor with any juices from the roasting tin and the garlic. Add the lemon juice, tahini paste and chickpeas. Season with salt and blend to a paste – add a little more oil if it's too thick. Scoop the hummus back into the pumpkin and serve with the peppers, breadsticks and pitta chips.

Baba ganoush & crudités

Ingredients

For the baba ganoush

4 large aubergines (about 1.2kg), pricked all over with a fork

zest and juice of 1 lemon

2 fat garlic cloves, chopped

3 tbsp tahini

4 tbsp extra virgin olive oil, plus a little extra for drizzling

For the crudités (optional)

4 large carrots, ends trimmed and spiralized into thick noodles

1 large cucumber, ends trimmed, spiralized into thick ribbons and patted dry to remove excess water

1 large courgette (about 145g), ends trimmed and spiralized into thick noodles

150g pack mixed radishes, cut into random shapes

Directions

STEP 1

Cover the hob in tin foil for ease of cleaning then put each aubergine on a single gas hob and cook, turning occasionally with tongs until the aubergines are completely charred and collapsed, this will take 10–15 mins. Alternatively, heat the grill to its highest setting, lay the aubergines on a baking tray and cook, turning occasionally, for 30 mins to achieve the same effect. While the aubergine is cooking, prep the vegetables if using.

STEP 2

Allow the aubergines to cool slightly then scoop out the soft flesh into a colander. Leave to drain for 30 mins to remove any excess water then blitz the aubergine along with the other baba ganoush Ingredients and some seasoning in a food processor to however smooth or chunky you like.

STEP 3

Spoon the dip into a bowl and serve in the centre of the vegetable crudités.

Stuffed cocktail eggs

Ingredients

12 medium eggs

6 tbsp bio yogurt

2 tsp English mustard

2 tbsp finely chopped parsley

For the salmon eggs

50g smoked salmon

sprigs of fresh dill

For the chorizo crumb eggs

25g chorizo, skin removed and finely chopped

Directions

STEP 1

Boil the eggs for 7 mins, drain and put into iced water to cool. Carefully remove the shells, then cut in half lengthways. Scoop the yolks into a bowl and mash with the yogurt, mustard and parsley. Spoon the mixture back into the eggs.

STEP 2

For the salmon eggs, top each with a strip of salmon and snip over some fresh dill.

STEP 3

For the chorizo version, fry the chorizo gently in a non-stick pan until the oil runs out and the chorizo is crisp. Scatter over the eggs when cool. Keep chilled until ready to serve. Will keep in the fridge for up to one day.

Pakora

Ingredients

1 green chilli, chopped

thumb-sized piece ginger, roughly chopped

1 tomato, roughly chopped

200g gram flour

1 ½ tsp chilli powder

1 ½ tsp garam masala

1 ½ tsp ground coriander

2 medium potatoes, peeled, halved and thinly sliced,
then halved into quarter moons

½ aubergine, thinly sliced, then halved into quarter moons

½ cauliflower, cut into florets

1 large onion, finely sliced

½ lemon, juiced

vegetable oil, for frying

chutney, to serve

Directions

STEP 1

Heat oven to 120C/100C fan/ gas 1/2. Make a paste by blitzing the chilli, ginger and tomato together, then set aside.

STEP 2

Mix the gram flour with the spices. Add all the prepared vegetables and toss in the mix. Slowly add 150ml water until the batter coats the vegetables – they should be well coated, but not swimming in it.

STEP 3

Add the tomato mixture and get your hands in there, mixing well until everything is incorporated. Add a little lemon juice and seasoning.

STEP 4

Heat the oil to 180C. Take a handful of the mix and squeeze it into a loose little ball, to ensure the vegetables stick to each other when lowered in the oil. Use a spoon to carefully drop the ball into the oil.

STEP 5

Fry for about 4 mins until golden and crispy, then taste to test for seasoning and consistency. You may also need to add a little water or gram our to the mixture at this point if your tester ball didn't hold together. Repeat, frying the remaining mixture in batches.

STEP 6

Drain on kitchen paper and keep warm in the oven as you go. Serve immediately with chutney.

Crunchy granola with berries & cherries

Ingredients

175g mixed nuts (pecan halves and peanuts in their red skins)

450g rolled oats

50g sesame seeds

50g sunflower seeds

125ml sunflower oil

100ml runny honey (try one of the lightly flavoured flower ones)

half a 170g packet dried berries and cherry

Directions

STEP 1

Preheat the oven to 190C/Gas 5/fan oven 170C. Halve some of the pecans, leave some whole. Mix with peanuts, oats, sesame seeds, sunflower seeds and a pinch of salt in a large bowl. In a jug, measure the oil and pour into the mixture, then measure the honey – it will slide out easily. Stir together with a fork to break up any big clumps of oats.

STEP 2

Pour on to a large baking tray with sides, preferably non-stick, in a thin layer. Bake for 20-25 minutes, stirring well at least twice and bringing the mixture in from the edges, until it is golden. Transfer to a large bowl and leave to cool.

STEP 3

Mix in the berries and cherries and serve with plenty of chilled milk.

STEP 4

Store for up to 1 month in airtight container.

Harissa sweet potato wedges

Ingredients

1kg sweet potatoes, scrubbed and cut into wedges

1 tbsp harissa paste

soured cream and chives, to serve

Directions

STEP 1

Heat oven to 200C/180C fan/gas 6. In a large bowl combine the wedges with the harissa. Transfer to a baking tray and cook for 40-45 mins until the potatoes are tender and crispy at the edges. Serve with soured cream mixed with snipped chives.

Crunchy cabbage salad

Ingredients

350g red cabbage, shredded

3 carrots, coarsely grated

20g pack parsley, roughly chopped

2 Cox's apples, quartered, cored and sliced

handful of radishes or 2 celery sticks, sliced

3 tbsp toasted pine nuts

1 tbsp pumpkin seeds

2 tbsp each sunflower seeds and linseeds

For the dressing

2 tsp grated root ginger

1 tsp clear honey

2 tbsp lemon juice

4 tbsp light olive oil

Directions

STEP 1

Prepare all the Ingredients for the salad and mix them in a large bowl.

STEP 2

Put all the dressing Ingredients into a small bowl. Season and whisk until slightly thickened. Pour over the salad and toss until evenly coated.

Rosemary, garlic & chilli popcorn

Ingredients

2 tbsp rapeseed oil

2 garlic cloves, lightly bashed

1 tsp chipotle or other chilli flakes

½ small bunch of rosemary, finely chopped

150g popcorn kernels

Directions

STEP 1

Heat the oil in a saucepan over a medium heat, then fry the garlic, chilli and rosemary for 2-3 mins. Remove from the heat, set aside and leave the oil to infuse for 30 mins.

STEP 2

Cook the popcorn according to pack instructions. Scoop the garlic out of the infused oil and discard. Toss the popcorn with the oil, then season and serve straightaway.

CHAPTER VI: BEFORE YOU GO, HERE'S A FINAL REMINDER!

Treating illnesses like cancer can feel overwhelming. It's common to want to do everything possible to help yourself feel better and recover as quickly as possible from CLL. While diet alone can't treat CLL, it can help support your health during treatment. Proper nutrition can make a huge difference during treatment and recovery and increase your overall quality of life.

More research is always needed, but your best option, for now, is to stick to a diet of lean protein, healthy fats, fruits, vegetables, and whole grains while taking steps to manage your treatment side effects.

You also need to pay close attention to food safety guidelines as you will be more prone to infection while under treatment. Talk to your healthcare team about ways to address the side effects of chemotherapy or other treatments.

www.ingramcontent.com/pod-product-compliance
Lightning Source LLC
Chambersburg PA
CBHW061038250726
48653CB00001B/147